Dental Practice Resource Group

Medical Emergencies In The

Dental Office

The Essential Guide

Case Based Teaching

© 2013 Dental Practice Resource Group

Dental Practice Resource Group

We are dedicated to providing easy to use tools for the thriving dental practice. Being there ourselves, we realize how difficult it is to accomplish patient care, administration and staff education simultaneously. By providing tools and resources, our team at Dental Practice Resource Group strives to lift the burden of fitting it all into an already busy practice.

This manual will provide both the templates that we use in all our operatories as well as discussion of some actual cases we have been involved with and those our medical director and consultant (M.D.) has been involved in over the last 17 years. Several of our staff have come to us from large multi-specialty practices in urban areas. The cases are both interesting and anxiety provoking. The goal of this manual is to instill a sense of comfort that your office can successfully manage the first few minutes of any medical emergency

The overriding key in any medical emergency is to remain in control of yourself and your team. Take a deep breath, have a staff member call 911 and never leave the patient unattended during an emergency situation.

This guide is just a small portion of the resources and training offered by Dental Practice Resource Group. Realize that sampling just a portion will not provide the whole flavor or experience, but will build confidence and knowledge when dealing with medical emergencies. Our M.D. Consultant has provided individual office training seminars that provides hands on experience utilizing mannequins, emergency equipment as outlined in this manual and practiced handling real scenarios.

We encourage your staff to read through the flow sheets and case scenarios several times. The goal of this manual is to provide both familiarity and insight into the process of managing the initial few moments of any medical emergency.

These templates (flow sheets) continue to serve our office and staff well and we believe they are the perfect tool to laminate and keep in every operatory. Reviewing them periodically at staff meetings is an easy way to keep everyone up to date. We suggest a minimum of biannual training refreshers sessions.

The list within is a suggestion as to what our practice group has found to be the minimum necessary equipment and supplies for a medical emergency kit. The templates below list common signs and symptoms but are not intended to be an exhaustive list of all possible presentations.

If interested in the video series that accompanies this guide, please contact us. We are working on a format to deliver those and allow easier access with the help of digital technology and file sharing.

About Us

Dental Practice Resource Group was formed with the sole mission of helping busy dental practices solve their practice related issues. Our team members have been practicing and collaborating on various projects over the last two decades and have come under the same umbrella a few years ago. We are very excited to have merged with Singularis Media Group and now have expanded our services. We have been using Singularis Media Group's web services for SEO, link building and video marketing for the last two years so the partnership was the next logical progression.

As busy clinicians it is very difficult to find the time to develop policies and procedures from scratch. Why reinvent the wheel? Dentistry at its core is the same wherever it is practiced; however, the nuances of practice management and marketing are what set apart the most successful dentists.

Our mission was to create a series of resources on a wide variety of topics specific to the dental office. Over the last year, we have been refining these resources and making them available to our fellow colleagues in the dental industry. We strive to make these resources valuable yet clean and simple. We have been told that their format allows for easy modification and customization based on the dental practice that utilizes them. With that in mind, we are making all of our resources available in a variety of formats (PDF, eBook, MS Word, RTF). Several of these formats lend for modification and can be tailored to any dental practice needs.

Our team is fortunate to have the input of a physician who shares a unique perspective on the issues at the crossroads of both dentistry and medicine. For that reason, we believe that our resources have a distinct advantage over what is otherwise available. Our business model is centered around a dental office and all of these resources and web-based strategies have been implemented in our own practice. Our team consists of dedicated health professionals who happen to be passionate about dental marketing and education.

Being a dentist and transforming lives (and smiles) has never been more rewarding. We know you will find value in this resource. Visit our website and see what else we have to offer.

DentalPracticeResourceGroup.com

Table Of Contents

MEDICAL EMERGENCY KIT AND EQUIPMENT

*Portable oxygen emergency tank-mask and nasal cannula

*AED

*Bag-valve-mask unit for positive pressure

*Preloaded syringe of Epinephrine (Adult and Child)

*Preloaded syringe of Benadryl

*Benadryl tablets

*Nitroglycerin tablets

*Oral glucose gel

*Albuterol inhaler

*Magill forceps

*Pocket mask for ventilation

*Short rigid board for CPR

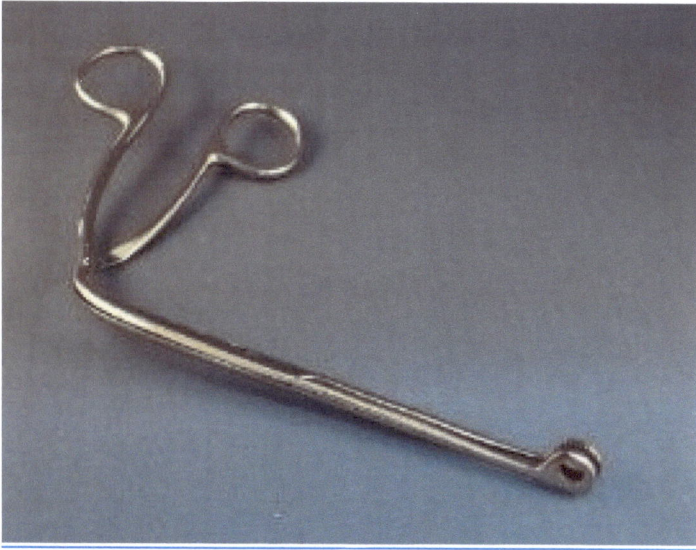

Magill Forceps for removing gauze and foreign material from a choking patient's throat.

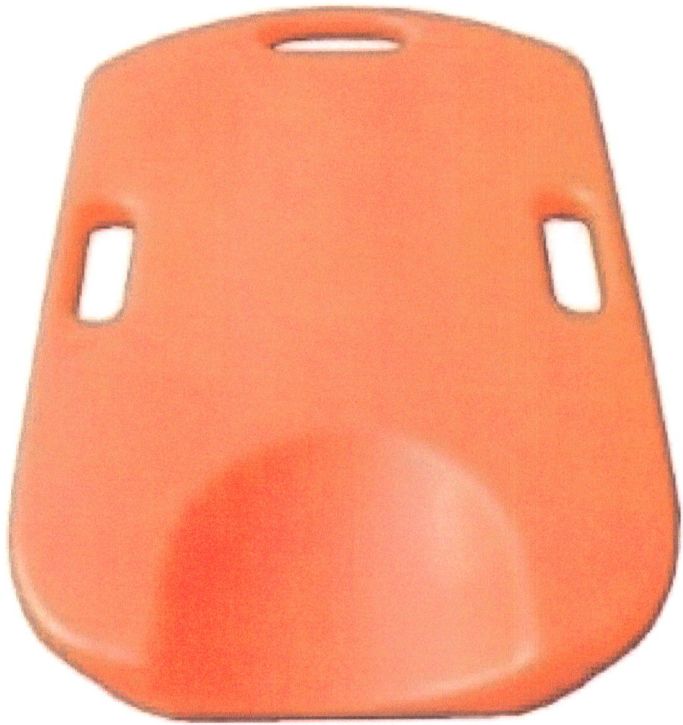

See larger image and other views

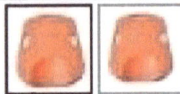

CPR board. It is very hard to perform effective CPR with a patient in a cushioned dental chair. This can also be used to help move or lift an unconscious patient.

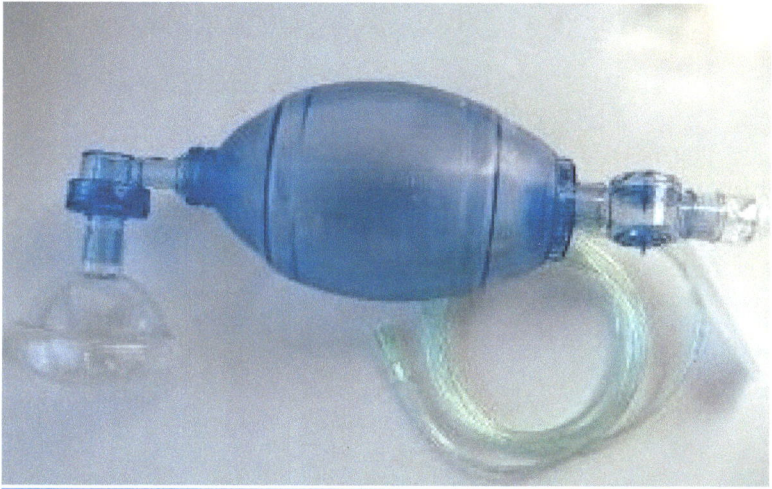

Bag Valve Mask to ventilate patient

Nitroglycerin tablets are a bit of an issue as their potency decays over time and there are some medical and physiologic issues related to using them. Benadryl, Pepcid and other antihistamines are readily available over the counter.

Glucose gel is common and a link to an example is provided above.

The Magill forceps is a must as we are aware of several cases from general dentists offices where patient choked on gauze and required expeditious transport to an ER to remove it.

Performing CPR in your office may be among the top nightmare scenarios. Without ridged support behind a patient, compressions will be ineffective. Above is an example of a short inexpensive rigid board. Annual CPR refresher training is a valuable component to maintaining competency among the dental office staff.

The above bag valve mask is also inexpensive and makes assisting or breathing for an unconscious or unresponsive patient much easier. It is also beneficial for those performing CPR.

An AED (automated external defibrillator) is a consideration, but if you life in a larger city, all EMS, police and fire carry AED. You may be fortunate to practice in an office or shared corporate office building that has them available. Make sure you have a basic understanding of their use. Most are foolproof with verbal instructions and pictures to guide the application and use of AED.

MANAGEMENT OF EMERGENCIES

1. Prevention is the best management

2. A thorough medical history and physical evaluation

3. T.L.C. Patient/doctor-assistant-hygienist rapport is the best insurance to avoid anxiety, fear and apprehension.

4. Appropriate and judicious use of pre-medication

5. Familiarity with medications (thorough understanding of patients medications, contra-indications and side effects).

6. Consultations, as indicated, with patient's physician.

7. Use of aspirating syringes for the administration of local anesthesia.

8. Advance preparation by establishment of a standard operating procedure for medical emergencies. The staff should be trained with specific prearranged duties. Dry runs are practiced periodically to insure office staff efficiency and competency.

9. Focus on care of the patient. Remember to breathe and don't panic!

Designate the following:

Emergency protocol Leader:

EMS Caller:

Emergency equipment 'go-for' Person:

Code Words:

Scenario:

Any unexpected emergency is chaotic at
the onset. Designating team members a
specific role in advance can provide
structure and add a sense of purpose to
the frenetic activity that ensues during
the first 15 seconds of any medical
emergency that occurs in the dental
office.

Emergency protocol leader – this
person is generally the dentist and will
guide the actions of the team members
and make the initial decisions in
management.

EMS caller – certain emergency situations should not require any second-guessing on whether to call 911. Patients with seizures, unresponsive, experiencing severe chest pain or any other condition that common sense implies the POTENTIAL for any life-threatening process needs to trigger a 911 call. Time is critical for certain conditions such as heart attack and stroke.

Emergency Equipment – this should be kept in a designated area and have a designated person assigned to retrieve the equipment. Keep everything together in one place. Use a box, plastic tub or commercially prepared kit. Keep it clearly labeled and easily accessible and make sure everyone who works in the dental office knows where it is kept. It should be checked monthly and after every use. Keep a written list of what is supposed to be in the kit and check expiration dates on any medications contained in the emergency kit.

Code Words - developing a set of simple code words provides a sense of clarity. Having a staff member scream or act out hysterically will create the wrong atmosphere and cause panic both among the staff, but also in the waiting room.

Use common sense when advising EMS which door to come through. If it makes sense and is easily accessible, have them enter through a back door, staff entrance or whatever door will facilitate entrance of their team and equipment. EMS will often bring a stretcher. Police or Fire department staff are often assigned to dispatch to medical emergencies in some cities and urban areas. So don't be surprised if some firemen in jump gear rush into your office.

Having them enter through the main waiting room obviously creates a sense of worry among the patients waiting. Care for the patient is paramount, but if possible and logical, direct EMS personnel to a quieter entrance and exit door.

SUMMARY OF COMMON DIAGNOSIS:

IF EVENT: is related to fear, apprehension and/or pain and occurs immediately following crisis event such as local anesthetic injection-think of simple syncope. (fainting or vasovagal reaction)

IF EVENT: occurs several minutes to ½ hour following a drug administration, and is accompanied with skin rash, hives, itching, edema, inflammation in nose and throat, labored breathing, bronchial constriction (heard as wheezing similar to a person with asthma), hypotension (low blood pressure) - think of allergic reactions. Evaluate rate of development and severity of symptoms. Allergic reactions can be mild or rapidly progress to anaphylactic shock.

IF EVENT: occurs several minutes after the administration of several carpules of local anesthetic and is manifest by either CNS stimulation or depression-think of local anesthetic toxicity. Major cause of death from lidocaine is cardiac (Ventricular fibrillation or arrest) followed by apnea. Lidocaine has direct effects on the myocardium (heart). Inadvertent injection into a blood vessel can result in quick and serious consequences. Major types of reactions from procaine, prilocaine, mepivicaine are respiratory arrest followed by cardiac arrest and death. Be prepared for convulsive seizure, vomiting and aspiration. It is unlikely that the toxic dose of lidocaine will ever be reached during a dental visit, but seizures are a sign of lidocaine toxicity.

IF EVENT: is related to a long duration or stressful appointment and develops slowly-think of metabolic events: hypoglycemia, adrenal cortical suppression, and hyperthyroidism. Stress of both physical and mental nature causes release of several stress hormones. These hormones can cause blood sugar to plummet and also affects other hormone systems (adrenal and thyroid) to a lesser clinically noticeable extent.

IF EVENT: is related to sudden onset of substernal pain with radiation to the arms, neck, or jaw and is associated with emotional or physical stress-think of cardiac cause (unstable angina / angina pectoris). The pain of angina should be relieved in 3-5 minutes with nitroglycerin. If it is not, think myocardial infarction (heart attack). Use extreme caution giving nitro to patients. If possible check a blood pressure first as certain types of heart attacks result in low blood pressure. Giving nitro will cause these patients blood pressure to collapse. Another point to mention: patients taking medications for erectile dysfunction (Viagra, Cialis, Levitra) should not take nitro if they have taking these erectile dysfunction medications recently as nitro can cause a serious drop in blood pressure which can be life threatening.

IF EVENT: is related to increasing labored breathing, swelling / edema, neck vein dissension - think of congestive heart failure. Certain patients with precarious heart function due to previous damage from heart attacks or chronic untreated high blood pressure can be quite sensitive to changes in body position. Many of these patients must sleep in a chair due to the redistribution of fluid that occurs when they try to lie down. In these patients the fluid that accumulates in the legs will redistribute towards the heart and lungs when they try to lie flat. This results in fluid building up in the lungs and a sense of suffocation and breathlessness (congestive heart failure). Ask patients with heart disease if they sleep in a chair or get severely out of breath when they lie down to sleep. They may be more intolerant of having the dental chair laid back very far.

Scenario:

Read though the above generalizations several times. Think back about patients you have had in the past with these conditions. If you ever have experienced a medical emergency in your office think back on what the clues were, the signs and symptoms the patient developed and how you and the other staff members reacted to the emergency.

DEBRIEF:

Debriefing is an important part of the process of learning and managing stress. After any emergency situation, take some time to discuss the case. While it may not be possible right then and there due o other patients and procedures being performed, set aside some time to discuss. Ask staff to write down some notes, thoughts and questions. Working though the case and your staff's perceptions will go along way to fostering an attitude of teamwork and make any subsequent emergencies go a bit smoother.

COMMON EMERGENCY TREATMENT:

<u>ABC'S</u>

<u>Airway Breathing Circulation</u>

1. If patient is awake and alert, allow patient to assume a position of comfort: Place patient in supine position if syncope occurs or is eminent. Lying down is the body's own protective

mechanism to restore blood flow to the brain.

 *Patients having a stroke, angina, heart attack, panic attack, or congestive heart failure but are still conscious may be more comfortable in an upright position.

 *Pregnant women in the late stages should be positioned on their left side, NOT supine (uterus compresses vena cava and decreases Blood Pressure).

2. Insure a patent airway (optional emergency tools, but can be as simple as opening the airway as taught in basic CPR). Simply asking the patient if they are "O.K.?" will provide information about their airway.

3. Administer Oxygen (separate Oxygen tank dedicated for emergencies).

4. Check the pulse and blood pressure

5. Supply a cool compress on forehead

6. Be prepared to call EMS and Provide CPR

7. The ABC's are the cornerstone of any emergency

> A = airway
>
> B = breathing
>
> C = circulation

8. Reassess the ABC's until the patient recovers or help arrives.

9. ABCD is an advance version of the above and adds D for disability. If the patient is not responding coherently, unresponsive or in cardiac arrest they are "disabled" and EMS will want to know this when the 911 call is placed.

Scenario:

The above is a common pathway for the initial seconds in any emergency.

Depending on what equipment is in your emergency kit, the steps may need to be modified.

NOTES:

Create a few written practice scenarios for your staff to work though. Have them verbalize what they would look for and what steps they would take to determine how the patient is doing.

CONDITION:

ANGINA (PECTORIS)

CAUSE: Insufficient blood supply to cardiac muscle, usually due to arteriosclerosis. May be precipitated by stress and anxiety.

Symptoms:

- Pain in chest

- Vital signs are usually good

- Pain may radiate to left shoulder, mandible or neck

- Patient may have a history of this problem. Pain usually persists for several minutes.

Treatment

1. Call EMS

2. Semi-recumbent position

3. Administer Oxygen

4. Check vitals-make sure systolic pressure is 110 or higher prior to giving Nitroglycerin

5. If this is the first time the patient has had chest pain we cannot be sure if the chest pain is angina and therefore Nitroglycerin may be ineffective or in some cases harmful. Make sure to establish if patient has had chest pain in the past and has used Nitroglycerin for this in the past before administering Nitroglycerin.

6. Always ask male patients about erectile dysfunction medications. Many will NOT include them in their medication history or list.

7. Reassure the patient

8. If patient's pain does not subside in 3-5 minutes, suspect myocardial infarct.

   **Never give Nitro if patient has recently used an erectile dysfunction medicine (within 72 hours as a generally guideline)

   **All patients with chest pain should be evaluated immediately in the ER. Call EMS / 911.

Scenario:

68 y.o. Mr. Smith is one of your most stubborn patients. He minimizes everything. Your staff notices that he seemed to be sweating in the waiting room despite a cool fall day. The front

desk staff said he told them he was taking a "mint" just before your assistant walked him back.

You note that he seems to be breathing a bit hard and still sweating. He says he was just rushing to get here on time. A quick review of his health history reveals a history of coronary artery disease.

He tells you to hurry up with the exam as his foursome is teeing off in 45 minutes and he hates to be late.

What do you do?

<u>NOTES:</u>

He confesses that he has been having chest discomfort for the last 2 days. Realize that many patients will not describe it as "pain" but rather use some other descriptor. The mint he took was actually nitro.

He tells you the nitro relieves the pain, but hasn't been helping today. You tell him you are calling 911. He sits up and refuses! Mr. Smith states he drove here and he will drive to the ER. Now what do you do?

It is within his rights to drive himself. Your duty is to express concern, state the risks and document that you discussed that with him and offered transportation via ambulance (EMS = emergency medical services).

Many patients state that they are not worried about themselves or getting into an accident on the way. One helpful way to frame the conversation is to remind them of children and families who may be injured if their medical condition deteriorates on the way. "How would you feel if you killed a child or one of your friends because you passed out on the way to the ER?" often causes patients to reconsider. Mr. Smith states he sees your point and agrees that an ambulance is the best mode of transportation. You and your staff keep him comfortable and the ambulance arrives promptly 6 minutes later to transport.

CONDITION:

MYOCARDIAL INFARCTION - Acute MI

CAUSE: Occlusion of coronary vessels

Symptoms:

- Severe pain in chest, which may radiate to the neck, shoulder or jaw.

- Palpitations

- Dyspnea (short of breath)

- Cyanosis

- Sweating

- Weakness

- Shock (low blood pressure, altered consciousness)

- Patient may have a feeling of impending doom

- Pulse rapid, faint or slow

- Patient may have feeling of being squeezed like having 'bands around chest' or elephant sitting on chest'.

<u>Treatment:</u>

1. Call EMS

2. Position the patient comfortably

3. Oxygen

4. Reassure the patient

5. If they generally take aspirin, administer 4 baby aspirin if no contraindication.

6. Consider nitro (read above intro on erective dysfunction and blood pressure issues)

Scenario:

One of your favorite patients is in today. She is also a close friend of your family. She needs a root canal on tooth #14. She tells you she is a little nervous, as it has been 10 years since she had any dental care. Other than being tired from what she said was a "poor night of sleep" she feels fine. She also mentions that she ate and took her insulin before coming to her appointment. She will be celebrating her 68th birthday in a few days and wants to get her tooth fixed before the party.

As you begin to sit her back, you assistant mentions that she seems to be sweating. The patient tells you that in addition to her tooth hurting, her jaw and front of her neck ache with pain radiating to her ear.

Do you proceed anyway or what else do you need to consider?

NOTES:

Given the age of this patient, diabetes (risk factor for heart disease) and her sex, she is having symptoms of angina and given the fatigue she may have already suffered a heart attack. Women may have different symptoms than men when it comes to heart disease. The neck and jaw pain are symptoms of an impending heart attack. Sweating is also a clue, but being that she is diabetic, it could be a sign of low blood sugar.

In either event you terminate the appointment and advise her that she needs to go to the ER. The best option is to call an ambulance. Understand that offering to transport her in your vehicle seems like a noble option, but may expose you and the patient to extra risk. What would you do if she became unresponsive while driving to the hospital? Thinking and planning ahead while considering the worst-case scenario is a way to avoid additional disasters.

She tells you that her doctor told her to take an aspirin every day, but she didn't today due to the dental appointment. You give her four baby aspirin as its antiplatelet effects have been shown to beneficial for patients having an acute MI.

EMERGENCY TREATMENT

CONDITION:

CARDIAC ARREST

<u>CAUSE:</u> May follow myocardial infarction (heart attack), respiratory obstruction or severe allergic reaction.

Symptoms:

- Unconsciousness
- No respiration, no pulse
- No blood pressure
- Pupils dilated
- Cyanosis (blue color of skin)

Treatment:

1. Follow CPR protocol –insure airway, breathing, and circulation (ABC's).

Scenario:

Your office volunteered to provide a morning of dental care in a local nursing home. All the patients are new to your team. The patient is a 91 y.o. male who tells you he is a marine and tough as they come. He needs a simple extraction of #22. Fortunately the nursing home has a small procedure room used for visiting doctors such as yourself, Podiatry and family medicine.

You inject a carpule of mepivicaine without epi. Everything is going fine when he slumps over and becomes unresponsive. You are in a special area of the nursing home set up for visiting specialists. What do you do?

NOTES:

Call a "code or code blue". Nursing homes are required to have call lights and many have "code" buttons to trigger a general alarm.

Assess ABC's and begin CPR if no pulse. Use a backboard if available to improve the quality of compressions. The nursing home will have a protocol for dealing with codes.

Realize that this patient may be a No Code. This means that a patient does NOT want any lifesaving measures or efforts. Unless they have a bracelet or it is clearly written on a patient's chart, assume that everyone is Full Code and begin the ABC's and CPR if indicated.

Continue performing high quality CPR with the assistance of nursing staff until the ambulance arrives. In this scenario the charge nurse arrives shortly after you begin CPR with a nursing aid and let's you know the patient is a "no code" and you can stop CPR. The charge nurse tells you the patient had several previous heart attacks. There was nothing you did to cause this nor could you have prevented it.

CONDITION:

HYPOGYLCEMIC SHOCK - LOW BLOOD GLUCOSE

CAUSE: Hypoglycemia, hyperinsulinism, excessive medication

or Fast. Can occur more often in diabetic with infection or a patient who failed to eat appropriately.

Symptoms:

- Nervousness
- Confusion
- Profuse Sweating
- Convulsions
- Coma
- Rapid Pulse
- Nausea
- Combative, Uncooperative, Abusive
- Stroke symptoms

Treatment:

1. Call EMS

2. Administer on full tube of oral glucose gel ([15mg glucose](#))

Scenario:

Shelly is a 32 y.o. mother of three. She is courteous, but always brings her three small kids who destroy your waiting room during her appointments. She has significant periodontal disease and decay due to several years of poor social circumstance. Fortunately she is now clean and sober. She was an alcoholic for 15 years, but the only reason you know this is that your hygienist was a high school classmate of hers.

She seems a bit "off", but that is not unusual as she is always late, somewhat unkempt and in a big hurry to get through the appointment.

She reports no other health history or medications. Your hygienist proceeds with scaling and root planning of one quadrant (SRP). During the procedure the patient begins to speak gibberish. Your brand new hygienist panics and calls for help.

What could be wrong? What is the next step and most appropriate action?

NOTES:

Low blood sugar can cause a range of bizarre and unusual behavior; it can even cause stroke like symptoms.

This patient has an odor of alcohol and is showing signs of low blood sugar (glucose). Given her erratic behavior and inability to speak coherently you assume she didn't eat and most likely took her insulin.

Get the emergency kit and administer the oral glucose solution. Understand that these patients can be combative and don't hesitate to call 911 for help. If you get her to take the glucose solution and she returns rapidly to a normal mental state it is important that food be consumed as well. The body will metabolize the glucose solution rapidly and without food and calories, the patient's blood sugar will began to drop precipitously.

The other challenge in this case deals with the odor of alcohol. Is the patient intoxicated? Many patients will learn to function with higher than legal levels of blood alcohol. With her small children in the waiting room, the ethical part of your brain should be sounding an alarm. This issue is complex but has presented itself several times in practice over the years. Having a strategy and policy to deal with the substance-abusing patient is paramount.

Calling 911 in this situation is the best option. The issue of medical impairment due to diabetes will be handled by medical staff and after pointing out the smell of alcohol and presence of children (who were driven by mom to your office) can be handled by law enforcement and social work in the ER setting.

CONDITION:

RESPIRATORY ARREST

CAUSE: Respiratory obstruction or drug overdose.

Symptoms:

- Change in pattern of breathing, which may progress to cessation of respiration

- No effort by the patient to breath
- Cyanosis

Treatment:

1. Call EMS
2. Supine position with firm back support or place patient on the floor.
3. Look in mouth to exclude foreign body
4. Insure patient airway
5. Oxygen, ventilate patient manually (one breath every 5 seconds)

Scenario:

Your 19 y.o anorexic college double major over achiever arrives for a root canal. She is hyped up as usual and requests nitrous as her former dentist always "gave it" to her. You are running 40 minutes behind due to some equipment problems.

The procedure is going off without a hitch when your assistant states that this is the "most relaxed" visit you have ever had with this patient.

You look up over the top of your loupes and notice that she seems way to "calm"! In fact it seems that she is barely breathing?

What are the first steps to take? What are to potential causes of this situation? What should you and your staff do next?

NOTES:

This patient has a psychological disorder and also uses sedatives to manage her anxiety and other personality disorders. She took an extra few doses of her Ativan (benzodiazepine / sedative) as she was worried and nervous about her appointment. The absorption occurred while she was waiting to start her appointment. The nitrous was just enough to push her over the edge.

You call a {insert your chosen code word here} and begin to assess the ABC's. She is still breathing, but slower and more shallow than normal. Your staff member responsible for calling 911 does so quickly but quietly so not to alarm the other 4 patients in the waiting room.

(Your partners will thank you for this if you work in a group setting).

Having practiced with the bag-valve mask, you and your assistant begin to give some gentle assisted breaths timed with her own breathing. You do so at a rate of between 12-16 breaths a minute. Her color looks good and she appears to be asleep.

The ambulance arrives through the back door with a police officer escort. An IV is started and the patient is placed on the ambulance stretcher and quickly taken from your office to the ER.

You receive a call from the ER doctor thanking you for the good job saving her life and reporting that in addition to the sedatives, they also found narcotic medication on her drug screen. She was admitted to the ICU and anticipated to make a full recovery.

Realize that patients may not be forthcoming in regards to what drug or how much they have taken. Use your best instinct and judgment if something does not seem right - you are probably correct.

CONDITION:

STROKE

<u>CAUSE:</u> Blockage of an intra-cranial blood vessel. Lack of blood flow to a portion of the brain.

Symptoms:

- Weakness, confusion, headache, dizziness, dysphasia, aphasia, varying amounts of paralysis, nausea, drooling, incoherent speech, unconsciousness, unstable gait.

- If trying to stand the patient may fall

- Vital signs usually remain good

Treatment:

1. Call EMS

2. Reassure patient

3. Leave patient in chair/slightly recline

4. Keep head elevated

5. Maintain airway

6. Oxygen and respiratory assistance if needed

Scenario:

After a grueling year of GPR, your residency is complete and you are back home to join your dad in his well-established practice. The experience and wisdom he shares is beyond any bond you had with your dental school instructors.

Your first year of practice is going great until your office manager interrupts a difficult procedure to tell you that your dad is acting strange.

You rush back to the break room and notice that his speech is not making much sense and he seems to be drooling. He is 64 and otherwise healthy.

Is this a test or is something serious happening before your eyes? What is the most important first step? What should you do next?

NOTES:

These are classic signs of a stroke. As with heart attacks, time is crucial when dealing with stroke symptoms. "Time Is Brain" is a slogan promoted by some health organizations for good reason.

Targeted therapies exist for patients experiencing stroke symptoms. Getting to the ER rapidly is key. Some medical therapies are not possible if too much time has elapsed from the onset of symptoms. The clock starts ticking from the moment the first symptoms appear.

Some patients may want to wait to "see if it gets better". It is best to talk them out of this and enlist family members, friends or call their personal physician to get reinforcement.

Being a person of quick action you help him to your car and fortunately you were able to get him to the ER in 10 minutes. The stroke team evaluated him, completed a head CT and administered specific therapies (clot busting drugs) that resolved the stroke symptoms.

Your father was back to work the next week without any deficits in part by your quick action in getting him to medical care quickly.

A word of caution about Aspirin

Stoke patients may qualify for potent thrombolytic therapy (clot busting drugs). Our office does not give aspirin to any patient with any neurologic symptoms. We prefer to defer that decision to the ER staff as some drug therapies are contraindicated if aspirin is given and it can increase the risk of bleeding. Not all strokes are caused by blocked arteries; some are caused by bleeding in the brain (hemorrhagic strokes). Aspirin in this setting would make matters worse. Most current protocols that utilized thrombolytics (clot busters) do not allow the use of aspirin in the initial treatment of strokes or for the next 24 plus hours (depending on the institution).

CONDITION:

SEIZURE / CONVULSIONS

CAUSE: Pre-existing seizure disorder or Reaction to drug (local anesthetic), substance abuse.

Symptoms:

- Signs of CNS stimulation (excitement, tremors, followed by convulsions)

- In Epilepsy (Grand Mal) aura (flash of light followed by cry from patient) will precede convulsion. (In some cases there is no warning)

- Absence seizure: staring or 'spacey'

Treatment:

1. Call EMS

2. Do NOT place anything in patient's mouth as this may cause more problems or injure the patient

3. Move anything out of the way that may hurt the patient

4. Patient may sleep deeply following convulsions. Be prepared to support respiration. Turn patient to the side to keep airway clear.

Scenario:

A 22 y.o. male with a known seizure disorder is in for a routine cleaning and wants to get a night guard made. Your assistant is in the middle of taking the impression when he goes "out".

She starts screaming and calling for help. Your staff rush to her aid and your are seconds behind. She missed the last meeting on office emergencies!

What do you need to do first? What about the impression tray and material? Should you pry the patients mouth open with something? What position should you put the patient in? What next?

NOTES:

This patient is having a seizure and it may take several staff to keep him in the chair. Move all equipment away from the patient. If you have any pillows, blankets or towels use these to try and pad the area around the patient.

Despite what is shown on TV, seizures do not result generally in wild flailing of extremities. Patients may have tonic-clonic movements where the arms, legs and head flex and extend in a rhythmic pattern.

Remove the impression tray as soon as possible. Having the material pass into the throat would be disastrous and block the airway.

Your staff already called 911 and the seizure stopped after what seemed like a very long 2 minutes. The patient is postictal. That means he is breathing, but unresponsive. With the help of your staff you position him on his side and use a gentle thrust of his jaw to keep his airway open. You assistant gently suctions the mucous out of his mouth.

EMS transports him to the ER where he receives and IV with additional anti-seizure medications. He fully recovers and returns to your practice 10 days later to finish the appointment. He apologizes and states that sometimes he is up late studying and forgets to take his seizure meds.

CONDITION:

ANAPHYLACTIC SHOCK

CAUSE: Allergic reaction

Symptoms:

- Respiratory and circulatory failure is progressive
- Itching of nose and hands, hives
- Flushed face
- Feeling of substernal pressure

- Asthmatic breathing, wheezing
- Coughing
- Sudden Hypotension
- Cyanosis
- Unconsciousness
- Edema (swelling)-face, lip, tongue

Treatment:

1. Call EMS

2. Position for Patient comfort

3. Oxygen, 10-15 L/min by mask or it may be necessary to ventilate patient manually with a mask or bag-valve mask

4. Check BP

5. Give Epinephrine (EPI pen: in leg or deltoid. 100lbs or less=child) IF:

a. Patient is exposed to known allergen AND

b. In respiratory distress, AND

c. Systolic BP less than 90

6. CPR if necessary

Scenario:

A 31 y.o. patient is in for what they state is the first dental visit they can ever remember. Her teeth seem to be in pretty decent shape despite the lack of formal dental care. You do detect several very small caries and she would like two of them fixed today.

You choose lidocaine 2% with epi. Everything seems fine except that she seems to be turning red and developing hives. Everywhere!

What is the cause? What are the first steps? What medication could save her life? What else could you give or do? What if the symptoms were mild? Or quickly resolved with treatment?

Another Scenario

It is a beautiful summer day. Your assistant brought her daughter with today, but plans to take her to the sitter during her morning break. The child is playing outside, but comes rushing in crying about a bee sting. Her lips are already swelling as well as her eyes. She seems to be having trouble breathing and starts to wheeze.

Do you have anything in your office to save her life? Do you or your staff know how to use it? Are there any training devices available? What dose or size do you use for this 7-year-old 60# child? What will happen if you don't act?

NOTES:

These are both straightforward examples of severe allergic reactions. These types of reactions can range from mild with just a little bit of itching or rash all the way to full blown anaphylactic shock with diffuse hives, extremely low blood pressure and shock. This condition will quickly lead to death if intervention is not provided immediately.

Epinephrine is the drug of choice for severe allergic reactions. Consider using it in any patient with severe diffuse hives, wheezing or swelling of the lips or tongue. Given the speed these reactions can progress, delaying intervention until help arrives may be too late.

The average ambulance response times vary by city. This information can be obtained from the ambulance companies directly or from the city directly who hires the ambulance company. Knowing this may give you some comfort, but it is just a generalized time. A major car accident may tie up several ambulances and the response time may be much greater than your office would like. This is another reason to develop a protocol to respond to severe allergic reactions.

Mild reactions can be treated with antihistamines such as Benadryl. Antacids such as Pepcid can also help, as they possess antihistamine properties as well. These are available over the counter and ask a pharmacist if unsure which possess antihistamine properties.

Epinephrine in the form of an auto-injector makes use in an emergency much easier. The syringes are prefilled with standard dose epinephrine and are available in two different sizes. The adult version for people weighting 75 kg or more and the Epi pen Jr. for those under 75 kg and children in general.

The only difference is the dose contained within each pen.

Understand that these are just temporizing measures. Any patient with severe allergic signs or symptoms needs medical attention. The effects of the above drugs are just part of the treatment equation.

Patients with severe reactions often require IV fluids and additional drugs to keep their blood pressure from plummeting as well as high dose steroids to blunt the allergic response occurring inside the body.

Any patient with symptoms severe enough to get an injection from an Epi pen needs ambulance transportation to the ER. That is a good policy we follow.

CONDITION:

URTICARIA, PRURITIS OR ANGIONEUROTIC EDEMA

CAUSE: Allergic Reaction

Symptoms:

- Urticaria (rash-usually red skin eruptions on face, neck, arms, hands)

- Pruritis (itching of face, neck, hands, arms)

- Angioneurotic Edema (swelling of lips, eyelids, cheeks, pharynx, and larynx, possibly leading to hoarseness, stridor or cyanosis)-requires ER visit

Treatment:

1. Benadryl: 50 mg orally every 6-8 hours

2. Benadryl: may be administered IM initially if problem is more severe. (Adult=50mg, Child=25mg)

3. Stop the drug in question

4. Contact patient's MD or an emergency room for follow-up care

5. OTC Antihistamine

Scenario:

The front desk receives a call before you arrive at the office regarding a patient you started on Amoxicillin yesterday. They state they are having some mild itching and notice a few bumps on their arm and a hive on their abdomen. Otherwise they feel fine and deny dizziness, swelling or any breathing trouble.

What do you tell them? Are there any medications they could take? Can you prescribe Penicillin instead or similar?

NOTES:

Mild symptoms such as itching and hives can be a sign of an allergic reaction. Common offending drugs include antibiotics and anti-inflammatory medications. Mild symptoms are not uncommon, but any severe symptoms should prompt following the above guidelines for severe allergic reactions.

Patients who have an adverse reaction to an antibiotic may have a much more severe reaction if exposed a second time to the same class of drugs. Avoid any other agents from the same family of antibiotics. Add it to their allergy list in the chart.

CONDITION:

ANESTHETIC REACTION

CAUSE: Excessive repetitive doses of local anesthetic; reaction to a component of the anesthetic.

Symptoms:

- Typical allergic symptoms – itching, flushing, hives

- Agitation fro low oxygen (methemaglobinemia from benzocaine)

- Dizziness

- Paresthesia (numbness and tingling of mouth)

- Twitching

- Grand mal seizures, coma & respiratory arrest

Treatment:

1. Reassure the patient

2. Local allergic reactions are usually due to ester class (procaine, novocaine, benzocaine). Less often to lidocaine. Give Benadryl for itching and hives. Swelling of lips or tongue – give Epi

3. May place oxygen and low flow (2L/min).

4. Severe reactions such as seizure are unlikely with the typical doses of anesthetic administered for most dental procedures.

5. Follow recommended dosing guidelines for the anesthetics of choice. I.e.: Lidocaine 5 mg/kg, Mepivacaine 4-5 mg/kg, Prilocaine 6 mg/kg, etc. Consult your preferred dental drug reference.

Scenario:

A 26-year-old presents for follow up of severe decay and two extractions. He was 20 minutes late and apologizes as he just came from his family doctor's office.

The typical amount of Lidocaine is used. The patient states that he feels dizzy 5 minutes after the injection was administered. He also complains of some palpitations and has some minor twitching developing. What could be happening? Any treatment immediately needed?

NOTES:

What the patient failed to mention is that his family physician excised several large moles at the appointment today. There was some bleeding afterwards and additional lidocaine was administered with epi to facilitate cautery and closure of the wounds left from the mole removal.

Your patient now has just exceeded the maximum recommended amount of lidocaine and is experiencing some symptoms of toxicity. Anesthetic toxicity can be severe and result in seizures. This would be a very rare occurrence with the standard amounts given in a dental procedure. In this instance the best option would be for this patient to be transported to the nearest ER and monitored for any worsening symptoms. There are treatments for severe anesthetic toxicity and consist of lipid emulsion therapy. This is usually a consequence of a regional block during a general or orthopedic surgical procedure.

Most of the anesthetic reactions occur due to a preservative such as paraben. Treat as a typical allergic reaction and transport to the ER if severe or anaphylactic symptoms occur.

CONDITION:

HYPERVENTILATION

<u>CAUSE:</u> Excess loss of carbon dioxide produces respiratory alkalosis. Panic attack. (Stress)

Symptoms:

- Rapid, shallow breathing

- Confusion

- Vertigo (dizziness)

- Paresthesia (numbness and tingling of extremities)

- Carpo-pedal spasm

Treatment:

- Reassure the patient

- Cold compress to forehead

- May place oxygen and low flow (2L/min). This acts primarily as a placebo

- Breath Into A Bag trick

Scenario:

Your 15 y.o. female patient seems to have had too much Mountain Dew at lunch. The afternoon was going great until she starts to breath rapidly and complains of tingling around her mouth and fingertips.

A pre-dental student is shadowing you today and asks if it is an allergic reaction to the local? How do you proceed?

NOTES:

The situation above represents hyperventilation and anxiety and not an allergic reaction. Rapid breathing blows off excessive carbon dioxide and this is the mechanism for the paresthesias. Your pre-dental student seems impressed with your explanation.

You provide reassurance and if that doesn't work the old bag trick. Having a patient breath into a bag traps carbon dioxide and helps to reverse the unpleasant paresthesias until the patient calms down.

She finally relaxes enough for finish the composite on #18 and you advise her on the evils of excessive pop consumption.

CONDITION:

SYNCOPE

CAUSE: Cerebral Hypoxia (Reduced blood flow to the brain); can be caused by stress, anxiety or pain (Vasovagal syncope). May be a sign of a cardiac rhythm problem.

Symptoms:

- Pallor (pale, cold, clammy)

- Anxiety

- Nausea

- Perspiration

- Tremors and convulsions (may occur if patient remains in sitting position)

- Loss of consciousness

- Variable pulse rates-fast to slow or slow to fast

- Pupils may dilate

- Blood pressure may be decreased

Treatment

1. Place patient in supine position (do not lower head below horizontal)

2. ABC's, vitals

3. Administer oxygen

4. Reassure the patient

Scenario:

After a lengthy SRP appointment, the patient states they didn't eat breakfast and is feeling ill. They seem a bit pale and ask to sit up quickly.

The hygienist puts the chair up and as the patient attempts to stand up, he falls back into the chair and is "out".

He is only 22 and has no health history, meds or allergies.

Is this serious and how do you treat it? How can you tell if something more serious is occurring?

NOTES:

Syncope or simple fainting is very common in the health care arena. Common causes are fear, dehydration and most commonly vasovagal syncope. We all know some patients, friends and family that pass out at the sight or even discussion of blood, etc.

Lie the patient back down and elevate the feet. This helps restore blood pressure and perfusion of the brain. The body has a normal protective response to passing out – assuming a horizontal position.

Provide something to drink such as water of juice and some crackers. Let the patient remain lying until the symptoms pass. Then slowly sit them back up a little bit at a time. Trying to rapidly sit them up or stand will likely result in another fainting episode.

If do not fully recover in roughly 10 minutes it may be time to consider other causes such as low blood sugar. This is likely the most common medical "emergency" in the dental office, but fortunately does not result in any long-term harm to the patient other than perhaps a little embarrassment.

What if the patient was 67 years old and complained of palpitations just before slumping over in your chair? This is likely a result from a serious dysrhythmia and could be life threatening. Syncope while seated or supine is always worrisome in an older patient. In this situation, first check the pulse. If present then have a staff member retrieve the AED and follow the instructions for applying and turning it on. Immediate Defibrillation from an AED is likely the most effective treatment to prevent death in a dangerous heart rhythm is still present in this patient. Your staff already called 911 right??

EMS
Preparing For The Ambulance

From the perspective of an ER physician, ambulance arrivals and departures are a normal part of daily activity *in the ER*. Having an ambulance show up at your dental practice is a whole different matter.

Issues to consider include:

- Which entrance is best for EMS (emergency Medical Services) to use

- Do you have a staff member to meet them and direct them to the patient

- Stairs, elevators and back doors

- What do you do with the crowded waiting room

- How to handle hysteria (family, staff and others)

- Remember HIPPA as your neighbors will often ask questions

- Getting back to work

- Debriefing your staff

These are all important and as a practice owner you will have to devise a plan that best suits your situation and office environment. If using a back door is easy and makes sense, then advise EMS and have a staff member direct them there. Avoiding a team of paramedics and ambulance stretcher wheeling through your waiting room should be a consideration. Obviously the care of the patient is paramount, but minimizing disruption to the front end / reception area is beneficial for a number of reasons.

Have a contingency plan for emergencies. What will you do with the next scheduled patient? Some patients or staff may become very anxious by an emergency situation. Do you have a plan to handle that?

If the dental practice is in an office building, neighboring businesses will often ask questions or comment on what they observed. Remember that patient confidentiality is key and HIPPA has mandates and stiff fines for violating privacy. What may seem like a harmless statement can come back to haunt. For example, the office CEO from next door asks what happened. Your staff says, "Grandma just got nervous and upset by the cost of her new crown, then passed out." This innocent statement is spread around the office complex and in reality the patient had a heart attack. How do you think she or the family would respond to the above?

"We had a ***medical emergency*** and it was handled appropriately" should be enough to suffice as an explanation.

SUMMARY

Some forethought and practice will go along way towards instilling some familiarity and confidence when dealing with medical emergencies in a dental office.

No one expects mastery and utter calm during these situations. Just step inside an ER and you will see flow sheets, charts, bedside resources and pocket guides in use during emergencies.

These situations are stressful even for those who routinely deal with them on a frequent basis. Stress causes errors and lapses in memory. Don't worry about it. It will happen to you as well.

Practice and discuss on a periodic basis and keep all current and new staff up to date.

We laminated our protocols and keep them chair-side in the same location in every op so that everyone knows where they are in any emergency.

All of our staff is familiar with the contents and the names of the devices in our emergency kit.

We have added the striped down versions of the protocols at the end so that you may modify to suit your individual practice needs and environment.

Additional Resources

We have included some of our most popular resources below. Please contact us if there is an area of your practice that could use a little assistance. Dental Practice Resource Group has many more resources and this is just a partial list.

We are a multifaceted group. We will listen to your needs and develop a creative solution that works.

Please visit our website for more information:

http://DentalPracticeResourceGroup.com

If you would like any of our resources in a different format such as PDF or MS Word please let us know. Some of our books and guides are already listed on the website but if you have purchased this comprehensive guide already, please let us know and with a copy of your receipt will be happy to accommodate your request for a different format.

1. OSHA Flow Sheet For Dental Offices

2. Sample Business Plan

3. Employee Review Checklists For All Positions

12.Link Building using White Hat Methods

www.ingramcontent.com/pod-product-compliance
Lightning Source LLC
Chambersburg PA
CBHW040512290326
41930CB00035B/5